Preface

Nursing is one of the most exciting professions today. Nurses are at the forefront of the healthcare industry. Nurses work to help patients cope with illness, prevent and disease promote health. Nurses are educators and advocates for their patients and their communities. Nurses collaborate with other healthcare professionals to provide quality and safe care to their patients. Essential to the nursing profession is the importance of respecting the cultural and human rights, the right to dignity, life and choice and the right to be treated with respect.

Gynecology and Obstetrics nurses specialize in the field of Nursing that emphasizes the care of women from puberty to menopause. Obstetric Nurses care for women during pregnancy, labor and childbirth. Gynecology nurses support expectant mothers before, during and after pregnancy and delivery care. They also care for women with problems with their reproductive system.

Unfortunately, the Nursing profession is not the same all over the world. Some nurses struggle to provide adequate and safe, quality care for their patients. In third world countries, nurses may even have to survive the cultural roadblocks that may hinder their practice.

Unlike the United States Nurses, Nigerian nurses encounter many professional and cultural obstacles in their profession. Before 1981, the Nursing in Nigeria was seen as a vocation and as unskilled. After 1981, the country started recognizing nursing as a profession. Unfortunately, most Nigerians still see the nursing profession as a "calling." Traditionally, Nurses were seen as a job for girls who are unintelligent, undesirable, and ugly. It was a job for women who could not get a husband. They were the servants and the mistresses of the doctors. As a result, nurses were not respected. Currently, with the demand for nurses globally, the image of nurses in

Nigeria is slowly changing. Nurses are still considered the servants to the doctors, rude and uncaring. They are not compensated well or well respected by their medical colleagues. Currently, the nursing profession in Nigeria is in the process of societal, professional and educational reform.

I have continuously questioned and compared the legal protection of women in the United States versus the plight of women in third world countries. For instance in Africa, women have continued to be subjected to inhumane and archaic treatments. Many injustices against women are rarely punished.

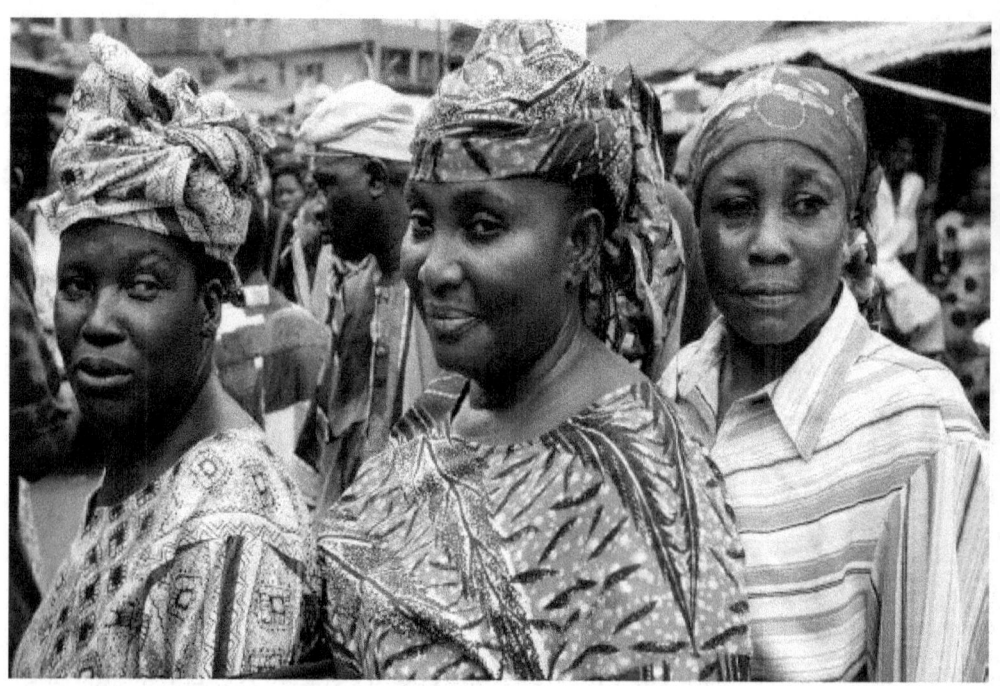

Courtesy of imgarcade.com -Traditional Nigerian Women

Contracts with women are rarely enforced. Women are constantly subjected to the inhumane crimes that are either overlooked or accepted as the norm. Many women are raped; girls molested and physical spousal abuse is rampant. Many indigent female patients lose their lives or the lives of their loved ones due to the negligence of healthcare providers and corrupt government officials. Women and children are more prone to poverty and aggravated crimes. It is common for women to die during childbirth or minor health-disease process. Until recently, many young girls still endure female circumcision for the benefit of their future husbands. The legal and equitable interests of the female relatives are rarely protected or enforced. Inheritance is only for the males in the family. As a result, male children are valued more than the female children.

Suspected adultery by a woman will not only bring chastisement, possibility of a divorce, and even death. Spousal support or child support is usually not an option. Some kids, especially the girls, are forced into early marriages or into child labor to provide for their families. If the woman seeks the court interference, she is faced with death or being maimed by her husband's family. Most women will either leave the country out of shame, fear or in worst situations, will commit suicide.

There is an expression that one man's meat is another man's poison. People complain the unfairness of their lives until they learn about other people's dilemmas. Some of the debatable topics of obstetrical nursing are intertwined with the controversial Nigerian cultural issues to showcase the plights of Nigeria nurses.

This story is about life lessons, survival and the resilience of a woman as she struggles to attain her cultural and human rights, the right to dignity, life and choice and the right to be treated with respect. Names have been changed to protect the privacy of others.

Life is full of lessons, are we ready to learn?

Nkechi

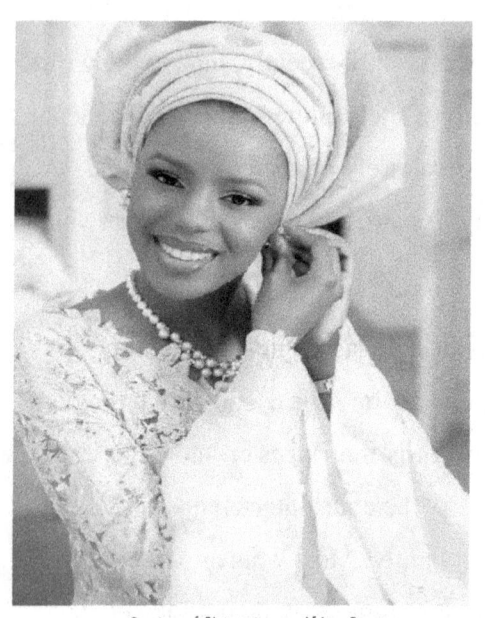

Her name is Nkechi (meaning for God). She is a maternity nurse, married with five children. She was a trained nurse who works and lives in Nigeria. She is just the same height as me, but slimmer. Her face is beautiful. Her eyes twinkled, and her perfect white teeth gleam when she smiles. Her brown complexion is polished with no apparent blemishes. Nkechi looks five years older than me even though we are the same age. She is the third wife of her husband.

In Nigeria, the incidence of child marriage is very rampant. Almost 45% of girls are married before their 18th birthday, and approximately 17% are married before they turn 15. These marriages are usually too much older men. Some of the factors that contribute to this practice include cultural, religious and social traditions. Recently, the Nigerian government passed a law that the age to consent to have sex is thirteen years.

Another factor is inadequate education. Education is a strong sign whether a girl will become a child bride. About 82% of women aged 20-24 with no education were married by the age of 18, as opposed to 13% of women who have finished high school. Finally, poverty is another strong indicator of the high prevalence of child marriage in Nigeria. Nigerian government is corrupted. This corruption is the primary cause of poverty in Nigeria. Many Nigerians are unemployed. More than 60% of Nigerians live in poverty.

4

Nkechi and I became friends when we were in high school in Nigeria. We both had dreams of becoming lawyers, marrying for love and living in fancy houses. However, after our final year in school, my parents sent me to the United States. Nkechi stayed in Nigeria because her family couldn't afford to send her to the United States or anywhere else to further her education. I remembered promising her that as soon as I could, I would send for her.

We kept in contact through letters. Six months after I left to the United States, Nkechi wrote to tell me that her parents were forcing her to marry a wealthy forty-nine-year-old trader from her village. Nkechi was sixteen years old. I wrote back and begged her not to do it. I urged her to run away. In between tears, she blurted that the man would help her family with her dowry.

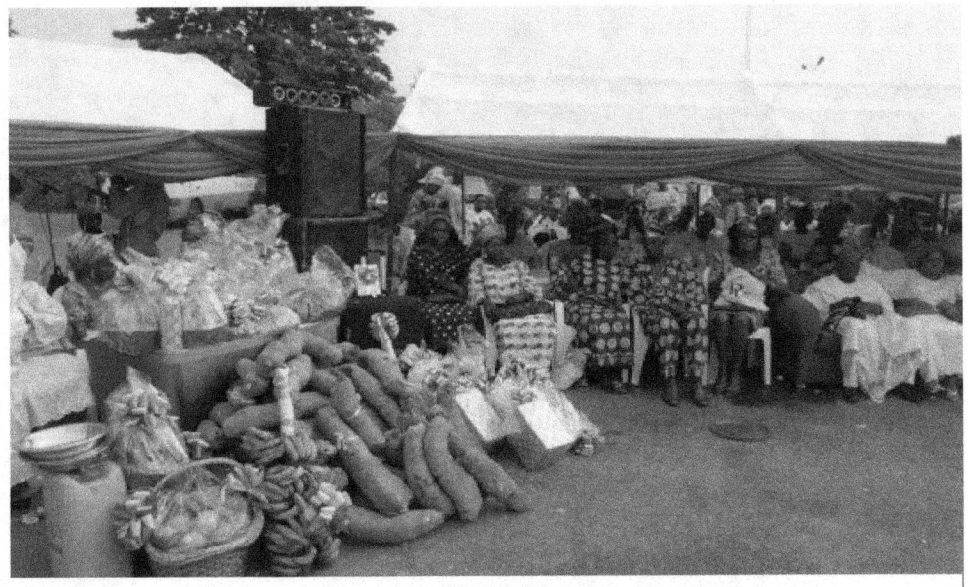

Courtesy of northoflagos.wordpress.com —Some of a Dowry for a Bride price

A dowry is a monetary price that a man must pay for marrying a woman in Africa. This monetary price includes money, food, clothes, lands, livestock and even cars.

In some tribes, this dowry may just be symbolic but in some tribes, it may be very expensive. The expense depends on the age, education and the family status of the bride-to-be. For instance, the dowry of a beautiful but poor 16-year-old girl with high school diploma will not be as expensive as the dowry of an ugly but rich 20-year-old woman with a college degree. As a result of the costly dowries, most men will see their wives as property. After all, the husbands paid enormously to acquire the wives.

2012 REVIEWED SAMPLE OF AN IGBO GIRLS BRIDE PRICE

	AA GENOTYPE	AS GENOTYPE	FAIR IN COMPLEXION	DARK IN COMPLEXION	SCHOOLED ABROAD	SCHOOLED IN NAIJA	TOTAL
UNIVERSITY GRADUATE	N150,000	25,000	200,000	70,000	500,000	200,000	
POLY GRADUATE	100,000	20,000	100,000	50,000	200,000	100,000	
COLLEGE OF EDU GRADUATE	50,000	15,000	10,000	8,000	100,000	50,000	
SECONDARY SCH GRADUATE	30,000	10,000	8,000	5,000	NILL	30,000	
PRIMARY SCHOOL GRADUATE	20,000	8,000	6,000	5,000	NIL	20,000	
UNEDUCATED VILLAGE GIRL	NIL	NIL	3,000	N1,500	NIL		

NOTE: Yams, palm wine, goat, cow, etc will be negotiated according to the girl's qualification, family's social status and beauty.
(Please calculate to the row and column that your prospective bride falls under and get the TOTAL)

Courtesy of omg.com.ng - How to calculate an Igbo girl's bride price

Two years later, she told me that she was pregnant with her second child and that her husband had agreed to send her to nursing school. She said that she was happy with her marriage because she could help her family. Also, she wrote that her husband and his two other wives were kind to her. According to her, she was helping her sister wives with raising their children. I was happy for my friend.

In the Nigerian tradition, men are allowed to marry many women as long as the men can afford to provide for the wives and the resulting children. Muslim

Nigerians can marry up to four wives. The church criticizes polygamy but some men still marry many wives. These men marry to show that they are rich. After all, wives are chattels. Some men will marry the first woman in the church and marry the rest in a traditional family. Some of these polygamous families are burdened with jealousy and violence. In some situations, the polygamous families tend to live together and share economic, family and social undertakings.

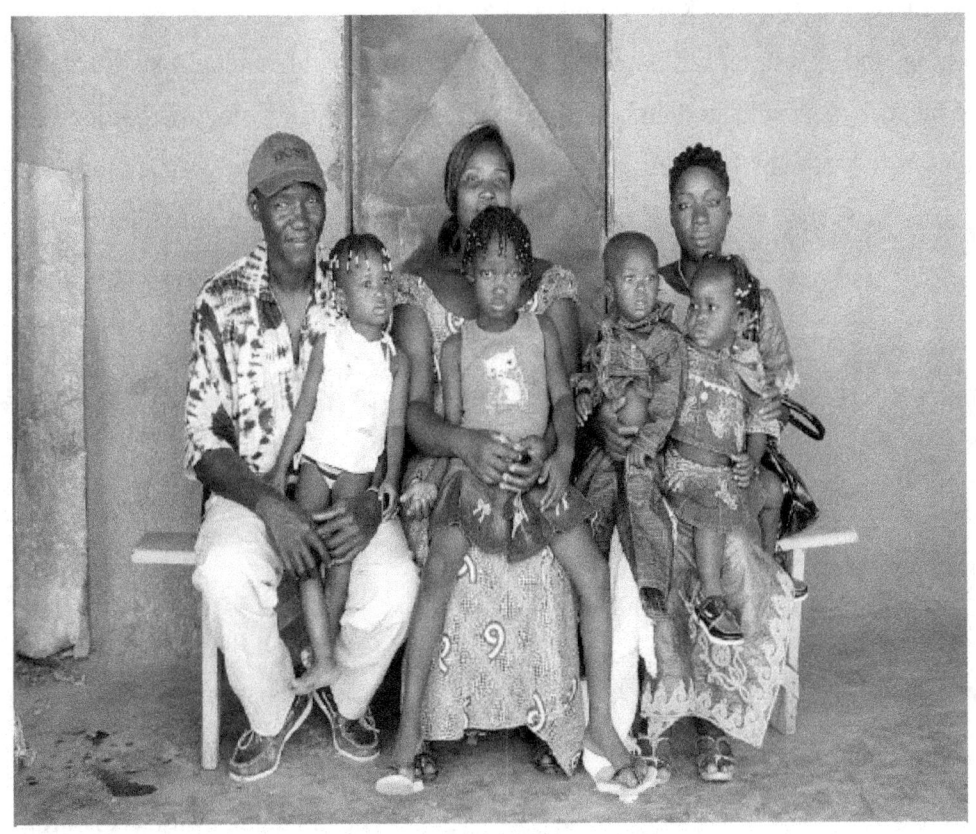

Polygamous family

After that, I wrote to Nkechi, but I never received any replies. I assumed that Nkechi was now busy with her studies and raising her children. I never heard from her again until I went home to visit my relatives sixteen years later. When she heard that I came back, Nkechi came to my father's compound to see me. At first, I didn't recognize her because she was dressed in a traditional outfit and carrying her son on her back.

Traditionally, Nigeria women would carry their children on their backs as a way of bonding with the child. This practice also allows the mother to do other things without worrying about the safety of the child. Most mothers would do everything with the baby at their back including cooking, washing clothes, cleaning the house, farming, and shopping. From a very young age, girls would be taught how to carry and balance their dolls and their siblings on their backs with a cloth tied around their waist. The baby benefits from this position because the sway of the mother's movements, body temperature and the mother's smell would not only soothe the baby but it would help to maintain the baby's thermoregulation. Most newborns would sleep and travel on their mothers', aunts', sisters' and in some cases even their older female cousins' backs most of their first year.

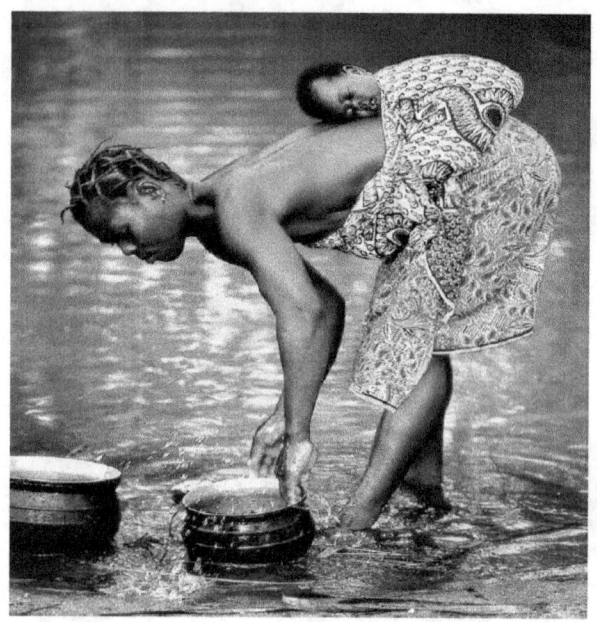
Courtesy of pinterest.com – A woman with a baby in her back while doing chores

Nkechi came running towards me with outstretch hands and calling me by my childhood nickname. When I was close to seeing her face and her angelic smile, I was overwhelmed with memories of childhood fun, girlish pranks and days of lounging in the sun and daydreaming. Nkechi and I hugged, laughed and danced. I held her hands for what seemed like hours. We were talking and laughing at the same time. For that moment, we were two giggling girls trying to catch up after sixteen years! Nkechi and I reminisced about our school days and our dreams. We shared stories about our families, about our friends and our dreams.

We sat under the shade of the mango tree in the sunny afternoon with a gentle breeze cooling us. I couldn't help marveling how our lives are the same. I realized that we have so many things in common. Nkechi talked about her experience as a nurse working in Nigeria. She described how Nigerian nurses struggle to provide care for their patients. I told her about my life as a registered nurse in the USA, and the challenges United States nurses grapple with every day. I complained about the health policies, the unequal access to care, the nursing shortage, the long 12-hour schedules, the rude doctors, the demanding patients and the seemingly lack of support from the Nursing profession stakeholders.

Nkechi smiled with a mischievous twinkle in her eyes. She challenged me to come with her to work for a day. I hesitated. I was thinking about the legal ramifications and the possibility that I might not enjoy myself – after all, I was on a vacation! Nkechi was adamant. She promised that I would have a unique experience and that we would spend more time together. I was sold! I accepted the challenge. I wanted to devote more time to this beautiful woman. The 16-year separation was brutal. I missed my friend! I agreed to go with her to work the next day.

Let's go to Work

As she was leaving, Nkechi promised to send me something that evening. I was elated. I couldn't contain my excitement. What would it be? Food? Pictures? My friend laughed. She told me to wait and see.

Later that night, her sixteen-year-old daughter arrived with a suspicious brown package wrapped in a yellow cotton cloth. Inside was a starched white nursing uniform with a stiff and faded blue apron. Wrapped in a white plastic bag was a white canvas shoe. As I lifted the dress, I saw something else in the package wrapped neatly in a silky white and blue scarf. I gently opened the scarf. Neatly tucked inside was a white, starched Nursing cap! I was elated.

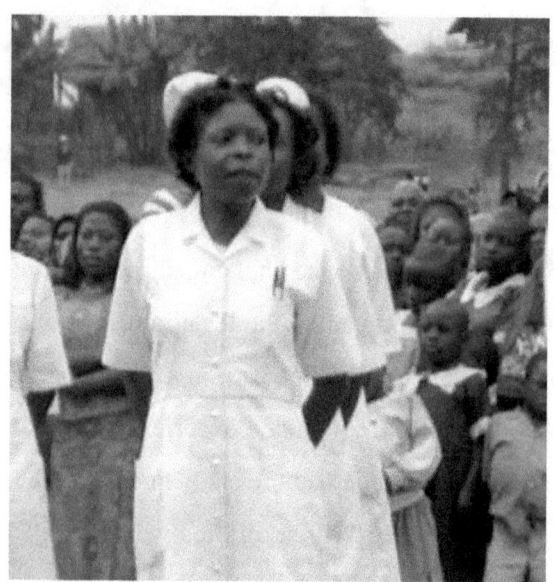
Courtesy of thenigeriangazette.com

The last time I wore a Nursing cap was during my pinning ceremony after my graduation from nursing school. I laughed out loud. I thanked Nkechi's daughter and sent her home. I hung the uniform in the closet and stared at it all night as if the uniform was going to jump off the hangar and attack me. I couldn't help wondering what if I should have declined Nkechi's challenge.

In New York, I work at a Magnet Hospital. I could wear anything to work. Since I insist on being comfortable at work, I never wore a skirt or a dress. My favorite Nursing outfit would be a white Jeans or pants matched with any color scrub pants and maybe a colored T- shirt or a Nursing scrub. When I became a Labor and Delivery nurse, the hospital issued me hospital scrubs – Green top and green pants. Due to the clientele of the hospital, the nurses were expected to be the poster model of customer service. Our uniforms are impeccably well-ironed and clean. We facilitate the labor and delivery of the crème-de la-crème of New York City. We had the best equipment, the most sanitary environment, the best doctors and the best of everything.

 So you can imagine how I felt the next day wearing a stiff white dress with blue apron and a nursing cap. I wasn't very happy about the cap. The cap had a mind of its own. It kept falling off my head. I was wondering how the nurses manage to care for their patients while making sure that the cap stayed perched neatly on their heads. By the way, the male nurses must have looked very silly wearing the cap. My mother explained that the male nurses do not wear the cap. WHAT!! That is sexism. Finally, my mom suggested pinning the cap to my hair with hair pins.

Once I dealt with the Nursing Cap problem, I was excited about the impending experience. I dressed in the starched white dress uniform. The hem was below the knees. I tightly tied the faded blue apron with two big pockets on my back. Next, I put the white canvas shoes, a pair of white socks, and pinned the cap to my hair. When I saw my reflection in the mirror, I couldn't help thinking what my Labor and Delivery colleagues would say if they see me garbed in a dress with an apron. I probably look like Florence Nightingale. When I came out to wait for Nkechi, my husband asked if I was going to a costume party!

Around 2:00 pm, Nkechi came to get me. She gave me an appreciative smile. She wanted to know what I thought about the uniform. I gave her almost twenty reasons why the dress should be torn, burned and buried. Nkechi was laughing so hard that tears were streaming out of her eyes.

I asked Nkechi where we would board the car. Nkechi looked at me incredulously. When she saw that I was serious, she looked me straight in the eyes and smiled. She told me in a firm voice that going in a car was out of the question. Cars would not be able to make it to the hospital. We had to take a motorcycle taxi until the cyclist couldn't go anymore then we would walk the rest of the way to the hospital.

I cringed! I've never traveled on a bike before. Sensing my anxieties, Nkechi promised that the trip would be safe.

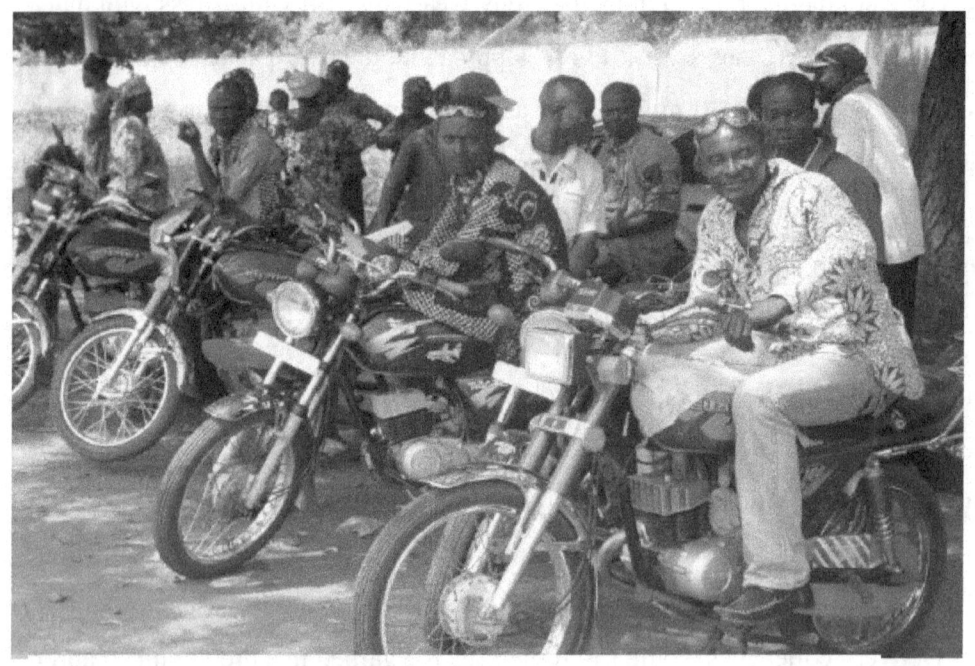
Nigerian Transportation

On our way to the motorcycle taxi depot, people were stopping us to exchange quick pleasantries with Nkechi. She greeted everyone back, dismissed an offer for payment for a recent circumcision she performed, gave some young women two minutes lecture about menstruation, administered an insulin shot to an old man with arthritis, and stopped to teach a young new mother how to calm a colicky baby. I was impressed! Nkechi was not paid for any of her services. When I asked her the rationale for doing all these services, she shrugged her shoulder. Nkechi explained that as a healthcare practitioner, she was obligated to help everybody who needs help. I was dumbfounded!

In New York, I remembered how one of the doctors was sued because he assisted in moving a hit-and-run victim from the road to the sidewalk. The woman sued the doctor for exacerbating her injuries. Even though the physician was acquitted of all charges, he was so distressed from the experience. It changed his life. The compassionate doctor became callous and distanced.

By the time we got to the bike cab depot, Nkechi seemed exhausted. She was sweating and moving a little slower than before. I asked her if she wanted to rest before we continue to our journey, but she flashed that incredible smile to reassure me that all is well.

The motorcycle ride was rather very fun. At first, I did not know how to sit. Should I straddle the driver? Then I saw Nkechi on her motorcycle cab. She was sitting sideways. The driver of another cab helped me to sit sideways, and I was instructed to hold onto the driver's midsection. I was petrified! I held onto the midsection of the driver so tight that he begged me to loosen my grip because he could not breathe. I asked for a helmet, and the drivers started laughing hysterically. When they finally calmed down and stopped laughing, one the drivers explained that they did not use helmets. WHAT!! I prayed all the way to the end of that ride!

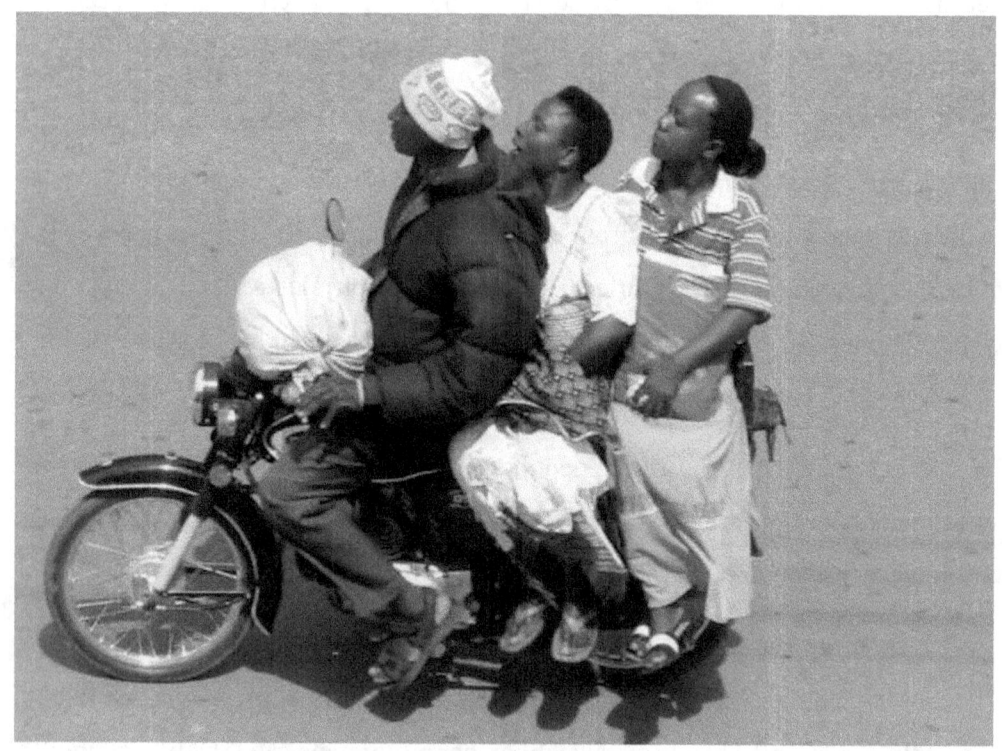

Courtesy of happytoursafrica.blogspot.com/public transportation in Nigeria

As we made our way slowly to the hospital, I realized why we couldn't take the car. The roads were full of potholes filled with mud and rainwater! We passed some brave drivers who attempted to swim through the holes. Their cars were buried in the mud with just the roof showing! Shortly after that, the motorcycles couldn't go any further. The roads became narrower and muddier. We got off and paid the drivers. By this time, my white tube socks and my white canvas shoes are stained brown with white patches. As we started walking towards the hospital, I regretted not wearing any pantyhose.

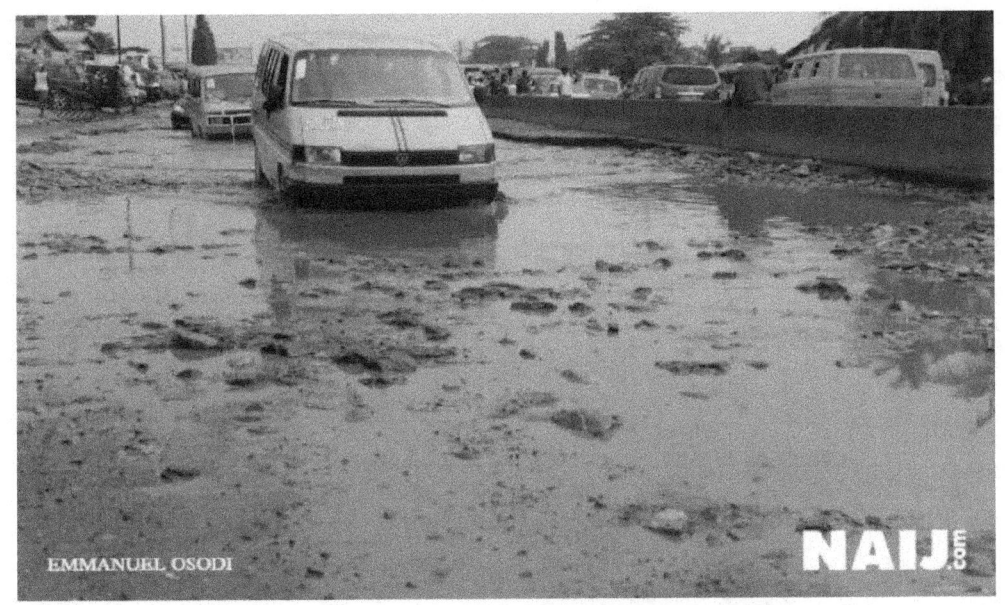

Nigerian Roads

The mosquitoes were everywhere. They bit me in so many places. I was practically scratching my legs sore by the time Nkechi stopped at a nearby bush. She searched around until she found a mysterious looking grass. She took some leaves, crushed it to a pulp and helped me to rub it over my exposed skin. The leaves smell like oregano with a hint of mint. Miraculously, the mosquitoes left me alone, but they managed to bit my ears and my fingers! I was a scratching mess by the time we arrived at the hospital.

Herbal medicine is widely practiced in Nigeria. Most Nigerian women learn from their mothers and grandmothers. Most people would rely more on traditional, herbal treatments more than the medical treatments. Some people will rely on spiritualists even to the detriment of their health. This reliance on alternative treatments may be attributed to poverty and inability to afford medical treatments and services.

The plight of African Women

Nkechi didn't speak too much on the way to the hospital. She seemed worried and anxious about something. When I asked her why she was so quiet, Nkechi told me an incredible story. Even though the weather was warm, I felt cold and nauseated.

Nkechi said that she might be pregnant again. I asked her why she couldn't use birth control. Again she laughed bitterly. She told me that the birth control pills that were sold at the pharmacy were not real. As for abstinence, she said that her

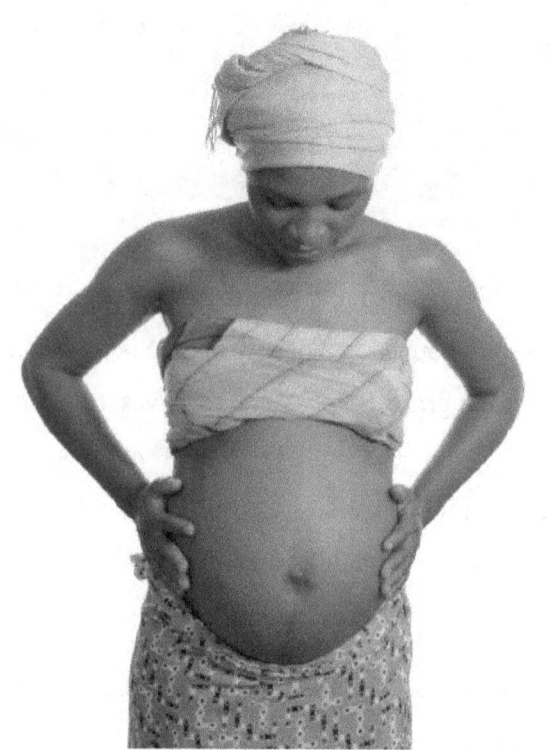

Pregnant Nigerian Woman

husband's sons and brothers rape her almost every night. She couldn't complain to anybody because they would kill her or rape her and her daughters. The sons may even force her to leave with her children. She stated that she was happy that her last child was a son. In Nigeria, women could not inherit the property of their husband except through a male child. A male child would ensure that Nkechi has a place in her husband's compound and would have rights to his properties.

Getting abortion was out of the question because it is illegal in the country. The quack doctors, who perform abortions, use unsanitary and dangerous procedures such as a metal hangar, mysterious herbs, and untrained medical practitioners to elicit abortion. Unfortunately, some of these women die from sepsis, imperforate uterus and hemorrhaging. Unmarried women who choose to carry the child to term would be ostracized and ridiculed, ostracize or even be subjected to violence. The unmarried woman would be considered as "whore" and as a "prostitute." Some women may be disowned because they would bring shame to their families. The children from these out-of-wedlock pregnancies would be considered as "bastards." This means these kids would never own or inherit anything.

As a result of this stigma, many of these unwanted pregnancies would end up aborted (albeit, dangerous procedures). Some wealthy families would send the girl away until she gives birth and the child would be placed in an orphanage. In some case, most of these babies would be killed or literally thrown away in the garbage or outhouses holes by their mothers. In the recent years, scrupulous organizations would recruit teenage girls and pay them from 100,000 Naira ($500) to 1, 000000 ($5000) to get pregnant and have babies for illegal adoptions, for black market sales and for rituals. A female child would be sold for 700,000 ($3,500) and a male child would be sold for 1,000,000 nairas ($5000) or even more.

As Nkechi talked, I felt sorry for her. I was also angry at a country that offers no protection for women and girls. Nkechi already had miscarried two pregnancies. She told me that she prayed for a miscarriage every day. Nkechi explained that the ordeal of providing for children was overwhelming. Her aged husband could not help because he became sick and bed-ridden. Nkechi was also worried that she might have contracted a sexually contaminated disease from her husband, his brothers and his sons.

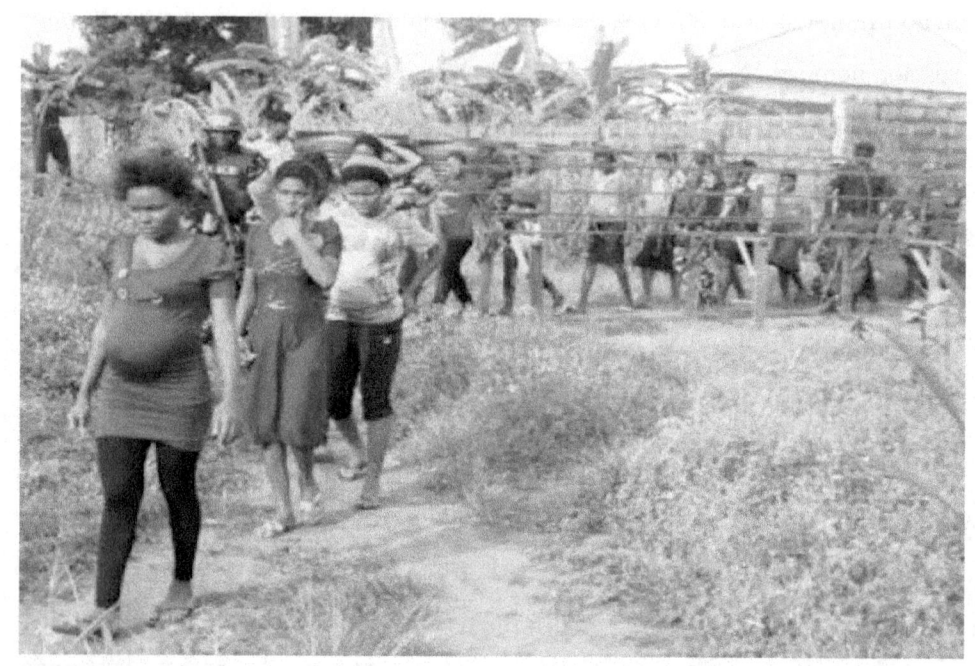
Courtesy of http://chukwudiiwuchukwu.blogspot.com - Rescues 16 Pregnant Teenage Girls

Most Nigerian women are not empowered to ask their sexual partners to use condoms or any other barriers. Most women who ask their husbands or sexual partners to use condoms may be killed or physically and emotionally abused. In fact, sex is not openly discussed. Without the support of some religious leaders, organization of these events proved to be a dangerous especially in Islamic areas where discussion of sex openly with women is a crime, and can be punishable by death. Finally, there is a cultural belief misconception and undertone about sex. For instance, some African women still believe that condoms will diminish the pleasure of the sexual act. Some African men perceive the use of condom as weakness and not manly. Since polygamy and even adultery is tolerated in some tribes and religions, STDs especially HIV have become very rampant in the heterosexual communities. Also, birth control methods are not readily available to some women because they are expensive or not available.

As we continue our tête-à-tête, I noticed that Nkechi was picking up sticks. Nkechi explained that for extra money, she would sell the sticks to the hospital's kitchen, and families of the patients. The sticks are valuable. They are used as fuel for cooking and for providing warmth. By the time we walked up to the hospital, we had about two bundles of sticks wrapped with banana leaf twisted into a rope.

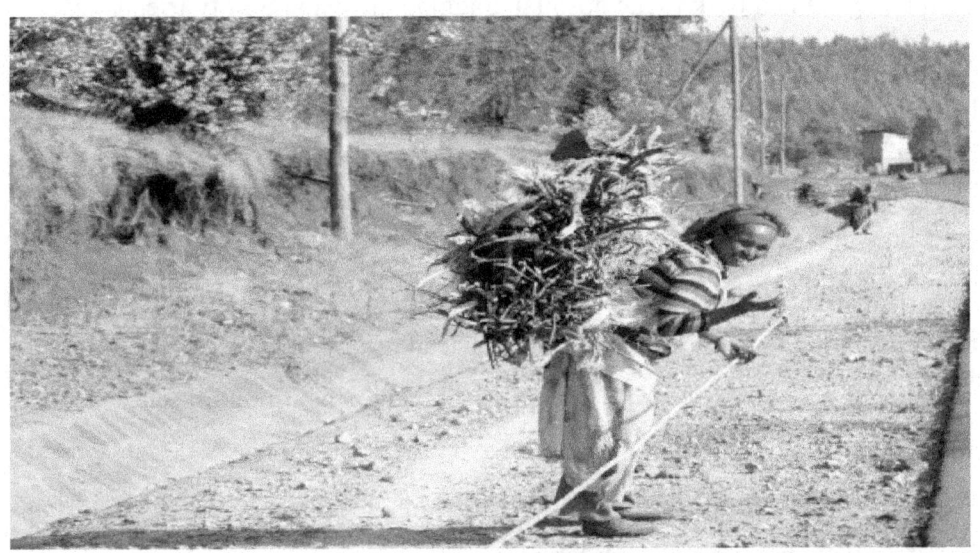
Woman carrying a bundle of sticks for sale

We took the bundle of sticks to the back of the hospital. An old woman ambled over to us. She examined the bundle of sticks as if she was reading an x-ray. Nkechi was getting impatient and was tapping her feet. The old woman looked up from the sticks and asked Nkechi how much she wants for the two bundles. Nkechi wanted 1000 Naira ($5.00). The old lady gave a weak and evil laugh then she blurted out that she thinks that 100 Naira ($0.50) was more than enough. Nkechi refused and started to collect the bundle to walk away. I could see that the old woman wanted the bundles of the stick. The woman then asked if 200 Naira ($1.00) will satisfy Nkechi. Nkechi adamantly refused and beckoned me to get the other bundle.

As we started walking away, the old woman sighed and gave her final offer, 500 Naira ($2.50). Nkechi stopped and dropped her bundle on the ground. I also dropped the bundle I was carrying. The old woman, muttering under her breath about the greed of young people, took out five wrinkled 100 Naira bills from her tied handkerchief and handed them to Nkechi. Nkechi thanked her while curtsying and quickly walked back to the hospital dragging me with her. My friend was euphoric about this. She carefully tucked the money neatly into her worn apron. By the time we got to the hospital, she was smiling triumphantly.

Nigerian Nurses are underpaid. The nurses are paid depending on their education and where they work (Private or Public institutions). Nigerian nurses make from 30,000 Naira ($150) to 350, 000 ($1750) per month. Unlike the United States nurses, Nigerian nurses are paid monthly instead of biweekly or weekly as their United States counterparts. These nurses must budget their monthly salary to ensure that it would last until the next payday. As a result, most Nigerian nurses may work outside of the hospital doing medical procedures such as circumcisions, teachings, petty trading and even farming.

To date, March 2016, one American dollar is equivalent to 200 Naira. Everything in Nigeria is very expensive especially the basic needs such as food, shelter, and sanitary pads, birth control and safety. The gap between the rich and the poor is very wide. There is no middle class. Most people would start indulging in illegal activities such as stealing.

Hospital or School House?

As we approached the hospital, I was dismayed. It was an old school house with damaged roofs. The walls were coated in cracked pale yellow paint and red dust. The shutters were painted dark sickly green. The grounds looked well kept except for the occasional pool of water here and there. There were mango and guava leaves scattered all over the ground.

Nkechi clarified that the town needed a public hospital so they started using the old schoolhouse until they could build a new hospital. She was happy that they converted the school house to a hospital because the next affordable hospital would be two hours away. As we approach the makeshift hospital, I could see that it was quite a large building with several extensions. Nkechi explained that including Maternity, the hospital has two other specialties – Medicine and Pediatrics.

On the south side of the hospital, there were a water well and some clothesline for drying clothes. Various types of clothes were drying on the line. Some people were washing clothes under the shade of the guava trees. There was a line of individuals waiting to get water. Nkechi explained that the hospital sold water from the well to the community. There was a low hum of the power generator. According to Nkechi, the generator supplies power to the well. Also, when the light goes off from the hospital, the generator would provide light to the hospital. Light supply is not consistently guaranteed to the hospital. At the northern side of the hospital, there was a garbage close to a brown wooden fence. Nkechi explained that all the waste is dumped at the site. The trash would be burned and eventually, would be buried.

At the back of the hospital, there was a building sectioned off from the rest of the hospital with the tall white fence. I could see three patrolmen in a security uniform.

According to Nkechi, the building houses the pediatric unit and the well-baby nursery. I asked why there was high security for the area. Nkechi then told me about an incredible story. This story gave me goosebumps until this day.

According to the story, approximately two ago, the hospital was attacked. Armed burglars invaded the hospital and made an abominable request. They demanded all the babies and the children at the hospital. When the staff refused, they gunned down two nurses, three mothers, one doctor and one orderly. They forcefully took ten newborns and seven toddlers. To date, those children are still missing. Nkechi speculated that the children were harvested for the black market for their organs. These kids would be killed and their organs exported to developed countries. Some of the children are also sold for black magic. After the incidence, the community decided to safeguard all newborns and children at the hospital.

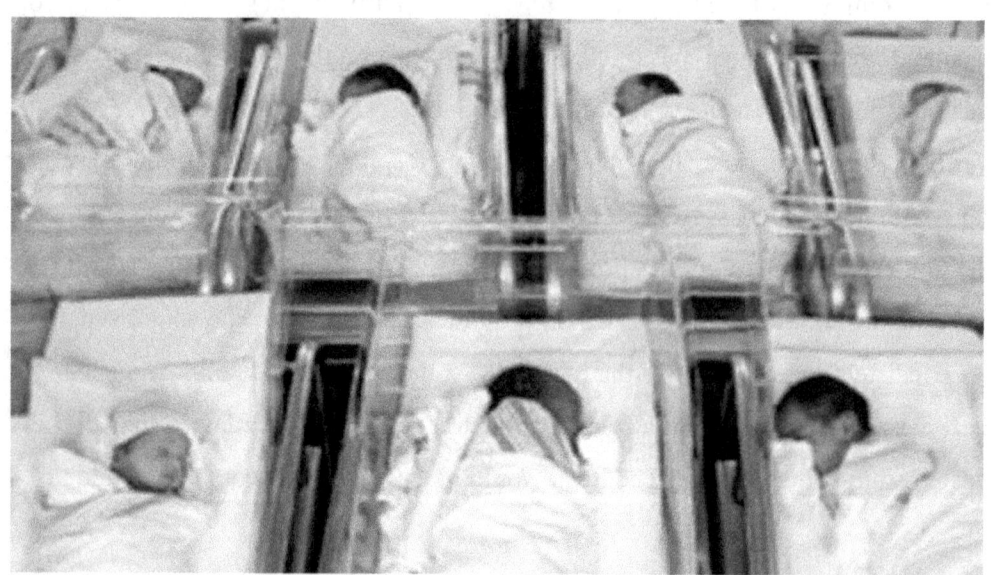

Courtesy of http://amazingstoriesaroundtheworld.blogspot.com - *Gunmen Storm Nigerian Hospital and Demand New Born Babies*

Most black markets would fulfill orders for hard to find organs such as heart, lungs, liver, and bone marrow by forcefully kidnapping of children from third world countries. Unscrupulous wealthy clients will pay well for these ill-gotten organs. The ritualists that practice black magic in Nigeria believe that human body parts have medicinal functions, offer protection from evil spirits, bring success, enhance prosperity and bring long life. Human blood, especially innocent blood and menstrual blood are seen as most efficient and very potent.

Ready, Set - GO!!

Nkechi hurriedly went inside. I followed her. I was intrigued by the smell of the "Hospital." The lobby smelled like a mixture of ammonia, medicine, bleach and another unidentified smell. Nkechi explained that the hospital custodians occasionally would use an astringent "Dettol" in their cleaning. The smell was overpowering. Many people sitting in the lobby of the hospital greeted Nkechi and curiously looked at me. I nervously smiled at them. As I followed her through the hospital, I became very nervous. What if I couldn't shadow Nkechi today? Where would wait for her? How could I get home? Would I be in danger?

I couldn't help thinking how different this hospital is when compared to the hospital in New York. In New York, the lobby of the magnet hospital has a very welcoming and comfortable ambiance. It is bright with welcoming lights. The Security guard standing by the entrance always has a neat uniform and an artificial smile. However, nobody in my hospital's lobby greets me as I walk into work. In fact, I try not to make eye contact with anybody in the hospital's lobby as I walk in!

I was amused how two nursing students passing us curtsied as we passed them! Nkechi turned around to make sure that I was still following her. I hurried up to catch up with her. She politely smiled at me, but I could see that she was irritated with my slowness. We stopped in front of red double doors. Nkechi paused and took a deep breath as if she was getting ready for a big audition. With a slight shrug, she fixed her nursing cap, wiped her sweating face with a starched white handkerchief from her pocket, and smoothed her faded blue apron with a worn and aged hands.

As I looked carefully at this great woman, I could see age setting in. She had dark circles under her eyes; there was a faint frown line on her forehead, and her mouth was pursed. I reached out and held her hands. She mistook my gesture as a sign of nervousness. Nkechi grasped my hands and did something that I always do before every shift. She closed her eyes and muttered a prayer. She whispered to me, "Remember that your hands are blessed and filled with the blessings of the Lord. Everyone you touched today should be blessed." I hugged her.

With a soft deep voice, she softly said under her voice "Ready?" I nodded and swallowed hard. I was not ready. In fact, I want to go back to New York right away. I didn't know what to expect. Behind those red double doors, I could hear women screaming in pain, babies crying and people yelling. I felt like I was going into the NCLEX examination room. I was afraid! What if I couldn't measure up? What if I was not trained well? What if…? I could hear the thumping of my heart. I thought to myself "Snap out of it. You've been through more than this before." So with a nervous tug at the white cap perched on my head and smoothing my blue apron with shaky hands; I reluctantly followed Nkechi into another world - into the maternity unit of a third world country!

The first thing that went through my mind as I entered the maternity ward was what my nurse manager always said during every staff meeting, "Be thankful that you are in a position to help somebody else." It was a dormitory type of ward. Women were lying on the bed, and all over the floor. Some of them were screaming for help, some were pushing unassisted, some were helping others to deliver, some were lying down in a pool of blood and amniotic fluid while cuddling or breastfeeding their babies and some were just lying on their bed sobbing or trying to sleep. There was no privacy. There was no fetal monitoring equipment. I saw few IV hanging freely without any electronic IV pumps.

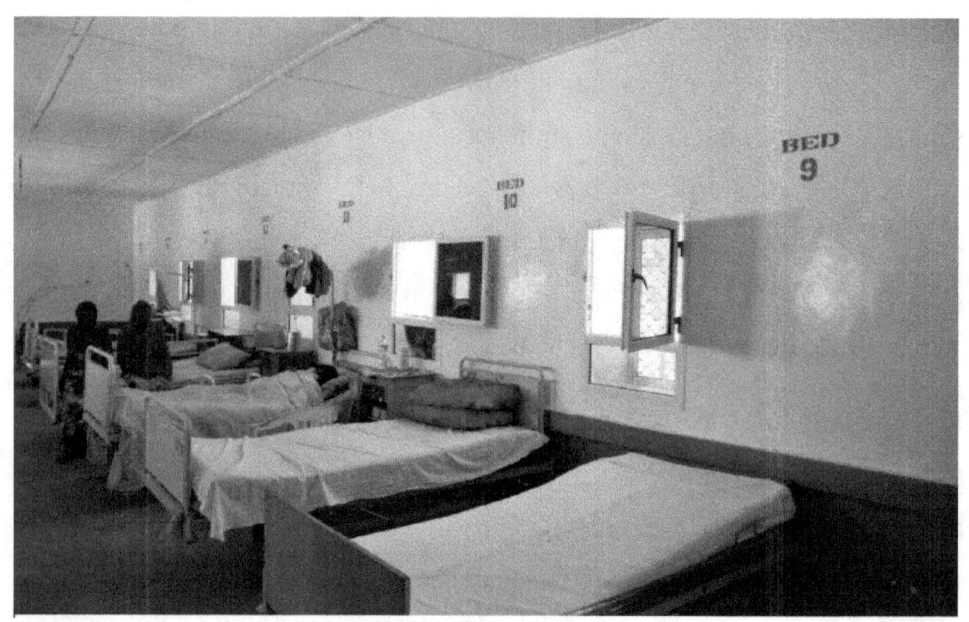
Dormitory style Obstetric ward

I saw one nurse with blood stained apron, profusely sweating, her cap slightly crooked. She was running from one bed to another attempting to help some women, scolding some to stop crying, and trying to bark orders at two young nursing assistants. One of the nursing assistants was picking up gloves and stuffing them in a basin. One young female doctor was at the desk arguing with somebody about needing the operating room to do a cesarean section. It was chaos!

Immediately, my nursing training went into action. I asked Nkechi what I could do to help. She looked at me quizzically and smiled.

"My dear, you can do anything you want to do. It seems that we will be the only people here today."

I was shocked. How can one nurse take care of more than a dozen laboring patients adequately? My friend must have guessed my puzzlement because she explained that she would use the female family members (males are not allowed in the delivery units until after the birth of the baby) and two women orderlies to accomplish her task.

I was relieved. I couldn't help thinking how my colleagues and I wrote a protest of assignment when we were short staffed by one nurse even though we still had six RNs for an eight LDRP suites and two operating room technicians. The nursing union would fight the administration for adequate staffing. The hospital will staff the unit per recommended professional standards.

Later on, Nkechi explained that most of the nurses had migrated to western countries in search of better life. Some of these nurses would migrate to the United States and the United Kingdom where they would make thirty times what they earn if they had stayed in their countries. Nkechi stated that if not for her husband and her aged parents, she would migrate to a western country with her children.

I followed Nkechi into the supply room. There were rows and rows of different sizes of gloves hanging on a clothesline. The gloves were secured with a peg. Nkechi explained that as a result of a limited supply of gloves, used gloves would be washed, dried and reused. Lined against the walls were cabinets and drums with names on it.

My friend explained that the patients bring their medical supplies because the hospital cannot afford to provide free supplies for the patients. The patients have to bring their sanitary pads, gloves, medications (RHogam, Pitocin, Colace, etc.), sutures, needles, antiseptic, and e.t.c. All these supplies including pain medications, antibiotics, needles, sutures could be obtained over the counter from a neighborhood pharmacy. I was distressed by this information because of the potential for abuse or misuse. Nkechi explained that the nurses would save the unused supplies for patients that couldn't afford the supplies, or the nurses would sell them for extra income.

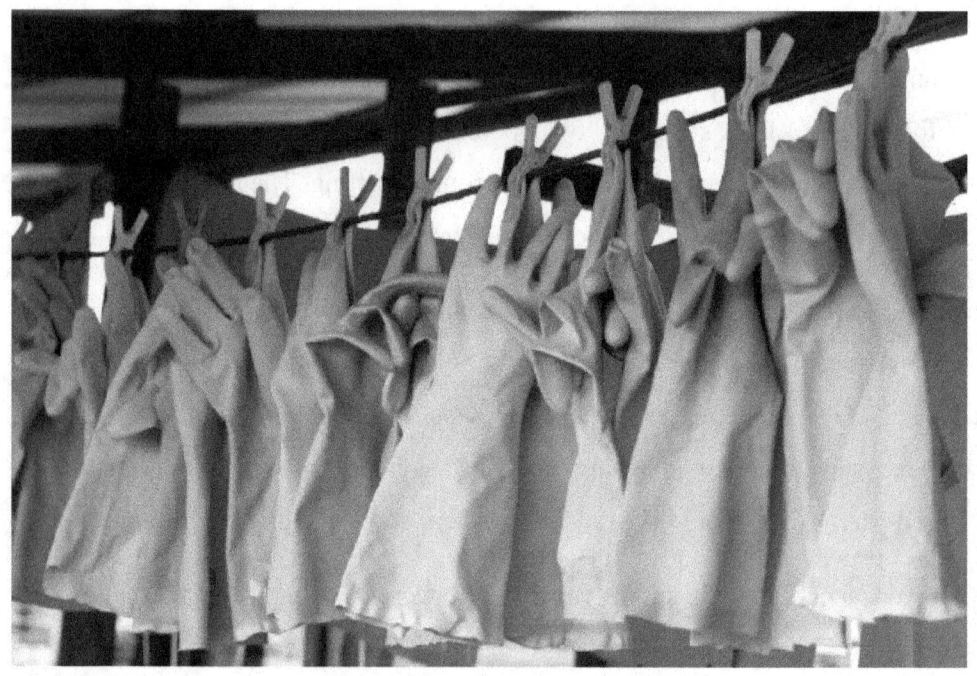

Courtesy of http://citizen.co.za - Gloves dry after being disinfected

We did a walking report with the morning nurse, Chinyere (translation -God's gift). She was so happy to see us that she gave us two-thumbs-up sign. I later learned that she has six daughters (3 sets of twins) ages two to ten years!! Armed burglars killed her husband on his way to work as a trader. So Chinyere was left to raise her children alone.

Every day after work, Nurse Chinyere would go to the nearby market to trade some fruits and vegetables to make extra money. Her relatives would watch her kids while she was working. Nurse Chinyere was saving money to migrate out of the country by herself or with her six children. Since she did not have a boy, Nurse Chinyere would never be allowed to inherit anything from her husband.

28

Life for Nigerian widows is appalling. Since women are considered the property of their spouses, these widows may be inherited by other male relatives of the spouses. Unfortunate widows may be prostituted, and in extreme cases, they may get killed. Some of the widows may remarry. However, if the widow decides to leave, they could not take their children. According to Nigerian culture, children belong to the man.

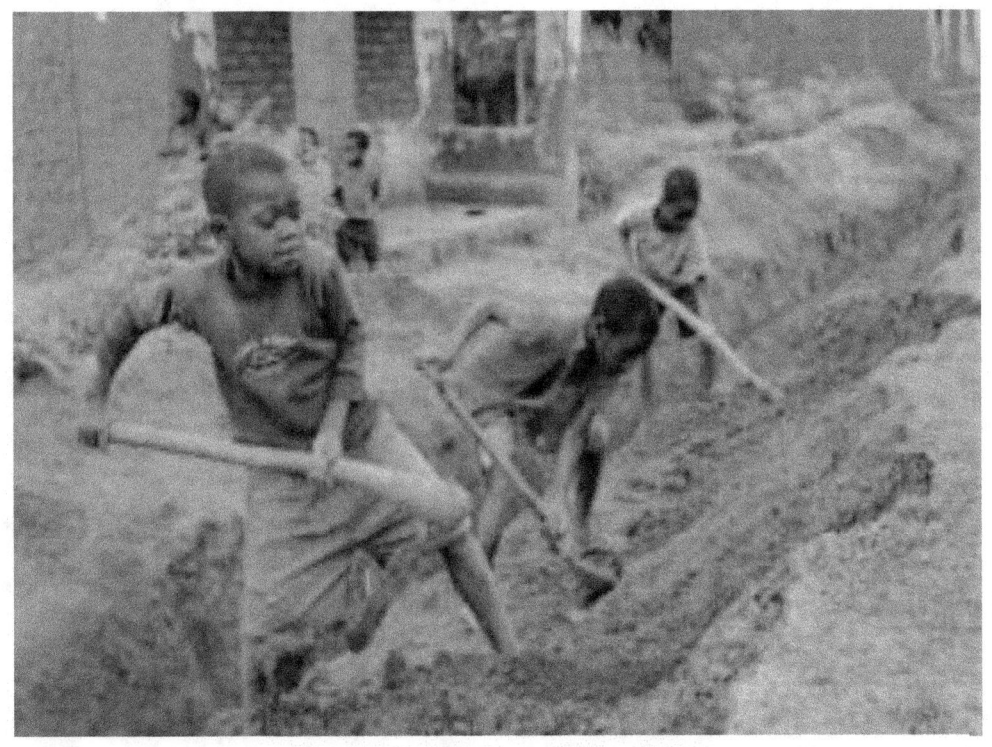
Courtesy of naija247news.com – Children Laborers

So the children would be raised by the families of their deceased husband! Sometimes, the children would be maltreated by the spouse's family. These kids may be used as child laborers or may even be kicked out to survive on the streets. Some of these children will beg, prostitute and steal just to survive. Child workers may get paid for 100 nairas a day ($0.50 a day). Also, most of these children would experience domestic violence and sexually abused and raped. Likewise, if the widows stay after the death of their husbands, they may be subjected to suffer emotional, financial, physical and sexual abuse from the male relatives of their spouses. For the sake of their children, some widows would remain single. They would stay with the husband's family and endure the difficulties.

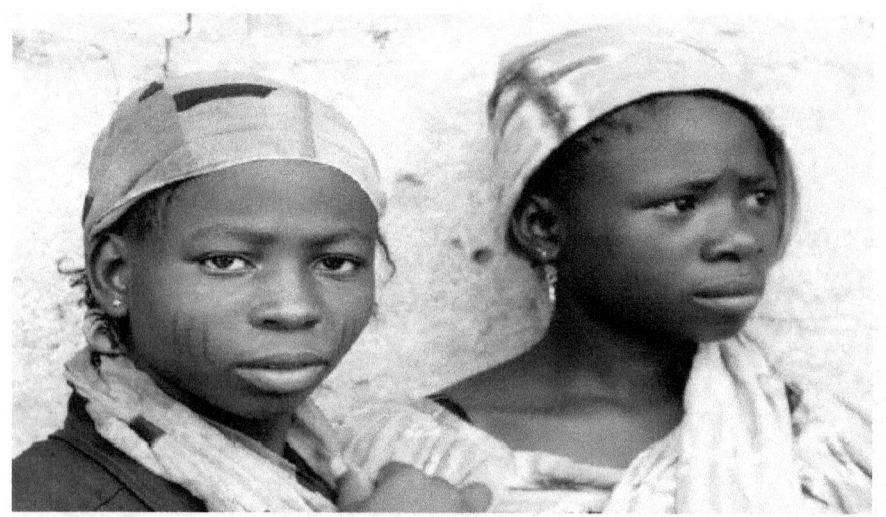

Courtesy of holgerawakens.blogspot.com-*Young Nigerian women rescued from human traffickers by Nigerian police*

During the walking report with Chinyere and Nkechi, the electricity went off. There was a blackout. It seemed as this was the norm in the hospital because the patients started lighting their kerosene lanterns. There are many power outages and blackouts in Nigeria because the country has inadequate infrastructure to handle the demand for electricity. Nigeria has very few power generating stations to put out enough power. The limited power is allocated. Due to the corruption of the country, wealthy neighborhoods and the towns would get electricity more than the villages or the poor neighborhoods. The outages could last from half an hour to months. Nigerians and institutions would get generators to supply their own electricity.

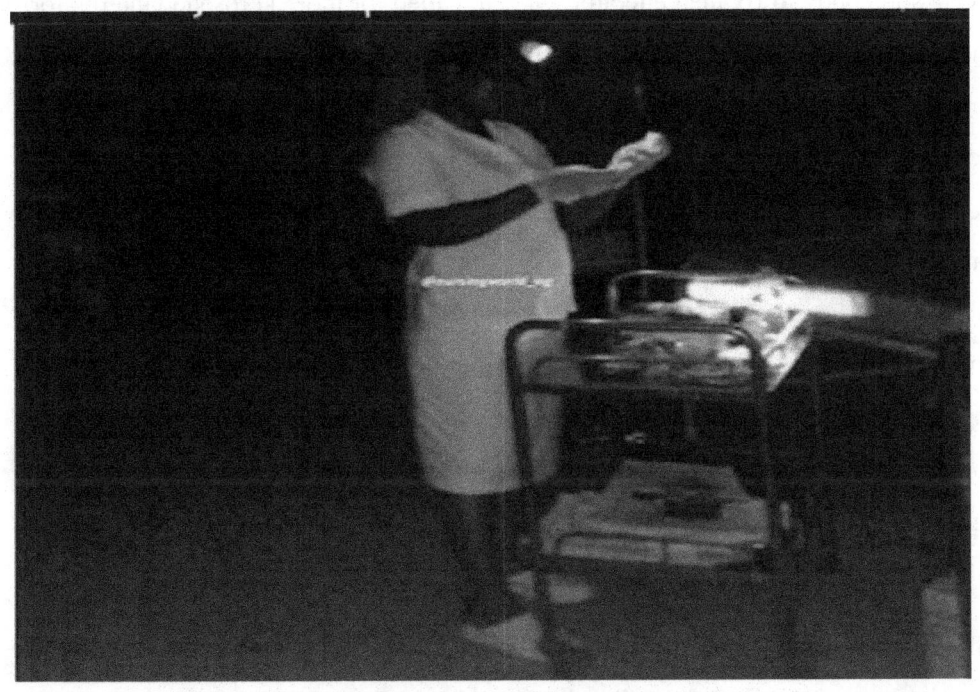

Courtesy of nairaland.com – Nurse using a flashlight to do patient care

The nurses quickly anticipated the physician's needs. Chinyere lighted a kerosene lantern and sent one of the student nurses to take it to the operating room. The young doctor started screaming for the generator because she was in the middle of a cesarean section delivery. Another doctor assisting with the cesarean section began berating the nurses for not anticipating the blackout. I was livid! Why would a doctor reprimand nurses in front of patients and other professionals? How come the doctor came out of the operating room to admonish nurses? I later learned that the second doctor was the attending doctor supervising junior doctors.

The two nurses did not respond to the ranting of the angry doctor. Instead, Chinyere sent an orderly to get the generator to start. The orderly came back and announced that the generator would not start. One of the orderlies was dispatched to get somebody to fix the generator. Nkechi called for more kerosene lanterns for the ward. Swiftly she took out torchlight with strands, attached it to her head. At this point, my eyes were popping out of my head. Chinyere informed the angry young doctor that he had to finish the Cesarean Section with the lantern. The doctor started chastising the nurses, the orderly and even the patient. He ranted and raved how impossible to work with incompetent people. Nobody stopped him or curtailed his unprofessionalism. He was so irate that he threw an instrument at the student nurse holding the lantern. The two nurses did something that made me bit my tongue so hard that it drew blood. The two nurses actually started apologizing to the fuming doctor! Chinyere curtsied while Nkechi promised to be better next time. After more angry chastisement, the doctor went back to the operating room. I was so upset and shaken by the whole incidence.

Nkechi explained that doctors still consider nurses as their subordinates instead of as colleagues. She told me that if a doctor walks into a room, the nurses were supposed to get up and offer the doctor the chair. Nurses were to carry out the doctor's orders without questioning it. If they defy the doctors, they could be dismissed. I was flabbergasted!

As if nothing happened, the walking report continued. At this point, my mouth was hanging wide! Since there was no running water, people were washing their hands in a basin standing next to the double doors. In addition to this community sharing of germs, flies were buzzing everywhere. I could just imagine what the infection control director at my hospital would say in a situation like what we saw. Apparently I was the only person worried because everybody else was not worried.

While getting the report on patient number two, the baby decided to come. Another orderly was sent to bring some gloves. The 20 y/o gravida four quickly pushed out an 8-lb baby out with the assistance from the two nurses. The patient was praised for her strength and efforts. After the delivery, my friend sutured a vaginal tear. The baby was whisked away by the orderly for a bath, and the relatives were instructed to clean the young mother up. Nkechi told the patient to take her two tablets of Panadol (acetaminophen). The patient was instructed to breastfeed the baby immediately and a family member was instructed to start fundal care.

Nkechi explained that the patient could not afford Pitocin and that the hospital did not have an unused medication. The whole thing took less than twenty minutes. We hurriedly finished the report so that Nurse Chinyere could go to her second job – peddling fruits and vegetables at a nearby marketplace. During all these delivery activities; the doctors were in the operating room finishing the cesarean section.

After Chinyere left, Nkechi and I quickly made our rounds. There were mothers to give encouragement with pushing, family members to support or throw out, babies to be checked, and blood pressure to be monitored (without the manometer), patients waiting to be sutured or assessed. During this running around I forgot where I was. I wanted to help each patient as much as I could. Mothers and their families were grateful. One patient clutched my hand after I had helped her to push. With tears in her eyes, she thanked me and blessed my future generations.

I was amazed that Nigerian nurses have a lot of autonomy. Nkechi was doing vaginal exams, rupturing amniotic bags, doing vaginal deliveries, suturing episiotomies, performing breech deliveries, administering medications without MD orders, and performing infant circumcisions. Nigerian nurses go through midwifery as part of their basic nursing education.

During one incident, the doctor was called for a prolapsed cord delivery. Nkechi had to finish the cesarean suturing – WHAT!! I was amazed and impressed. When I raised my objections, she looked at me dubiously and asked,

"Do you see any doctors here?"

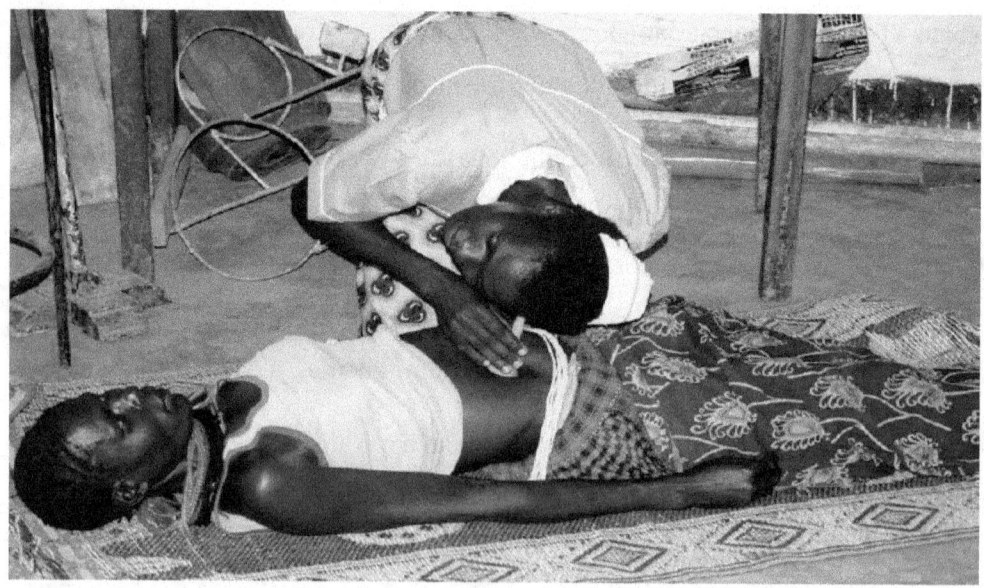

Courtesy of www.thelondoneveningpost.com – Nurse listening for the baby's heartbeat on a pregnant mother lying on the floor

She was right! The doctor never came back. We heard that since they do not have electricity, the doctors had to transfer the patient with cord prolapsed to another community hospital thirty miles away. Unfortunately, the baby died in utero. The mother died two days later. The unfortunate death of the woman was not surprising because the patient was carried on a stretcher to the bike depot. Then the bike took the patient to a bus station. The patient with a prolapsed cord took the bus to the hospital!!

Unlike developed countries, the mortality rates in African nations are appalling. In 2013, the Nigerian government reported more than 11,000 deaths in 3 months. According to the WHO, the African and the Caribbean countries have the highest rate of maternal mortality. Per WHO, the major contributing factor of maternal deaths is a preexisting health condition exacerbated by pregnancy. For other African countries, other contributing factors are governmental and social issues. Medication, efficient obstetrical techniques, and proper handling could easily prevent the high mortality rate of African women.

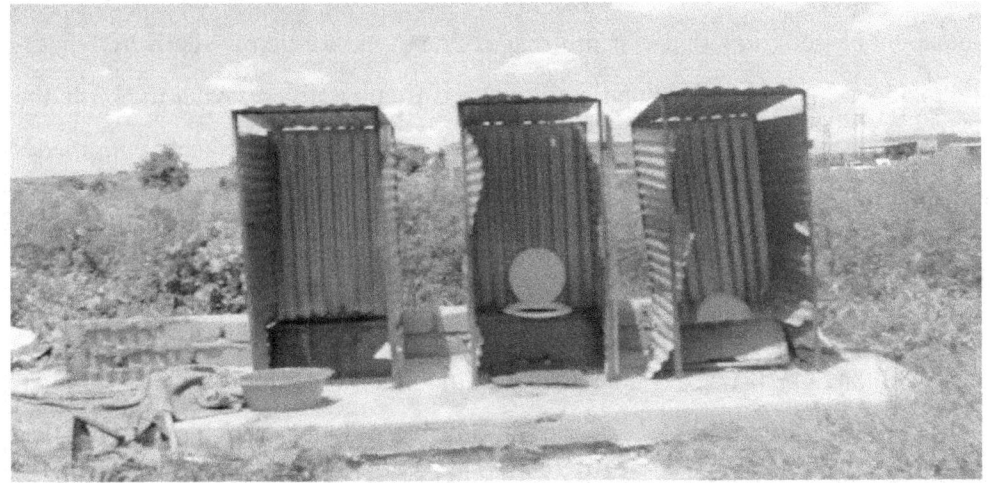
Courtesy of www.miyela.org – Outside outhouses

We did not get food or snack break except to stop to use the outside restrooms. The restroom was an outhouse with a hole in the ground. Over the hole, there was a wooden chair with a hole in the middle. On the rafters, lizards were resting in the rafters. I was uneasy every time I had to use the outhouse. The outhouses have been known to collapse and people have accidentally fallen in or drowned.

The air in the hospital was humid. We were sweating like hogs. As for me, the mosquitoes came back in full force to contribute to my agony. I gave up trying to kill the bloodsuckers. By the end of the day, I became used to the bites.

Surprisingly, I could not feel the bites anymore. My guess is that my body became used to the mosquitoes bites.

At the end of the shift, we have delivered ten babies. Two preterm babies were sent to the NICU. We did ten episiotomies and vaginal repairs. We discharged eight mothers to the recovery area. However, we admitted six more mothers. In the midst of all the mayhem, Nkechi and I managed to console three frustrated doctors, communicated with countless of concerned family members, and transferred one patient to the teaching hospital because of placenta accreta. Later on, we heard that the patient passed away due to hemorrhage. One of the women we delivered that night had a total vaginal infibulation. It was a difficult delivery. After the birth, the woman begged to have her vagina sutured back the way it was. Nkechi complied and sutured her back.

Infibulation is the most extreme of female circumcision. It is known as type three. Type one is the removal of the clitoris. Type two is the removal of the inner labia and the clitoris. Type three is the removal of the inner, outer labia and the complete suturing of the vulva while leaving a hole for urine and menstrual blood. After the procedure, the circumcised girl's legs will be bound together to enable the healing of the vagina.

After marriage, the hole is pierced with the husband's penis or with a knife to allow for sex. During delivery, the vagina would be cut open for the birth (deinfibulation). After giving birth, the vagina will be sutured back (reinfibulation). People who practice female circumcision believe that it is a way to maintain modesty and chastity in women. Some African tribes believe that uncircumcised women will poison their husbands during sex with their clitoris or become promiscuous. To secure wealthy and reputable men for marriage, families would insist on circumcising their daughters.

In actuality, the reason for circumcising women is a means of controlling women's sexuality and freedom. It is a method of ensuring that a female would tolerate the sexual abuse from men. If sex is seen as only for procreation and not for enjoyment, women would tolerate the man's excuse to bring in more women into the marriage. Women circumcision usually would cause difficult delivery, bleeding, chronic pain, infertility, voiding, painful sex, organ damage, incontinence, infection, trauma, obstetric fistula and chronic infection.

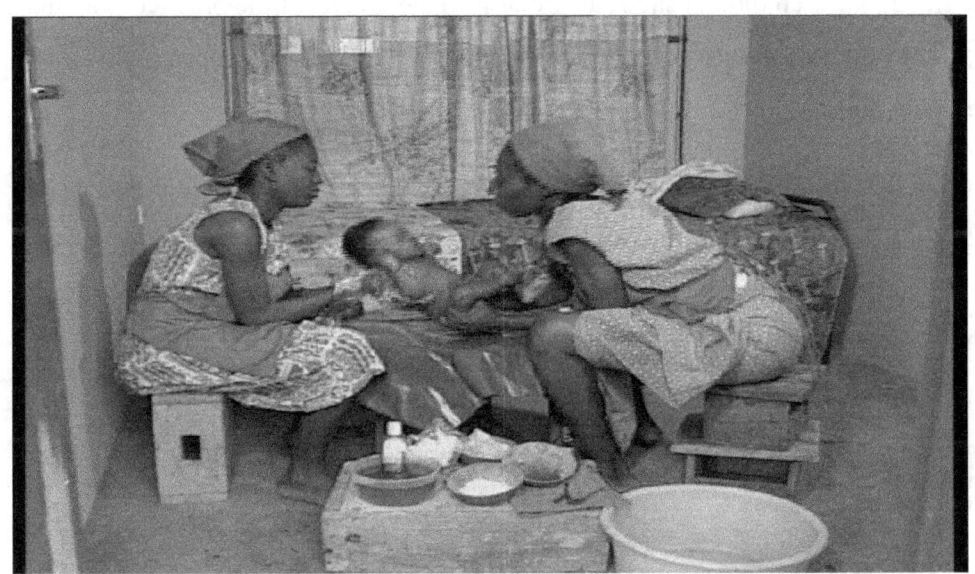

Courtesy of protumat.blog.com – Female circumcision

After the delivery, I told Nkechi how distressed I was about the circumcised vagina. Nkechi listened attentively as we were trying to do a Leopold maneuver on a 15-year old. After we finished and reassured the young mother that her baby was in the right position to come out vaginally, Nkechi and I went outside for a quick bathroom break and fresh air. Outside the unit, Nkechi told me that she was forced to practice Type-four vaginal mutilation at the persistence of her husband.

Type-four vaginal mutilations involve the forceful use of the non-medical procedure to mutilate the vagina. This mutilation could be scraping of the clitoris, tightening of the vagina, piercing the clitoris or labia. The side effects of these procedures include abrasions exposing the woman to STD, infections, bleeding, trauma, allergic irritations, Keloid formation, painful urination and sexual intercourse, irritation, obstetric and gynecologic problems, condom compromise and even psychological problems. Nkechi told me that after every delivery, her husband insisted that she use a combination of herbs to tighten her vagina. Nkechi admitted that even though she is aware of the side effects of the practice, she must also obey and satisfy her husband. She looked so helpless. I reached out and gave her a big hug.

During the shift, the electric power was not restored, and the generator was never started. All procedures were done with candles, kerosene lamps, and flashlights. I saw some patients slapping off buzzing mosquitoes. At one point we ran out of gloves, so we had to use the recycled ones drying on the windowsills. One of the orderlies was kept busy cleaning and powdering some soiled gloves for the oncoming shift. The exhausted orderly was also manually washing, sterilizing pieces of equipment and sharpening scalpels.

When the night nurse, came at 11:45 pm, I was so ecstatic to see her. I hugged her. I was exhausted, hungry but surprisingly very satisfied!

Is it over?

I looked at Nkechi and smiled. Our uniforms were dirty, and our caps were crooked. The faded apron seemed like a butcher's apron. The starched white uniform was wrinkled and stained. The white canvas shoes were now brown and pink with a little evidence of white.

The obstetric ward was now quiet with only two mothers in active labor. We quickly gave the-end-of-the shift report to the matronly nurse with a kind face, Nurse Obioma (Good Heart). She has been a nurse for forty years. According to her, she would never migrate to the western countries. Her four children live overseas, and they are living very comfortably. Obioma lives with her retired schoolteacher husband and plans to retire next year. Obioma complained that she wished she could retire now because she has arthritis and pains.

Unlike the United States, there are no social services available for retired and old people. There are no social security benefits or even Nursing homes. Retired workers depend on their pensions for survival. Sometimes, the pensions are owed by the government for an extended period of times. These retired workers would depend on their adult children and relatives for survival. Unfortunately, the adult children and families may be in the same quandary and would not be able to offer any assistance. These people who worked all their lives would struggle to survive. Some of them would die from acute illnesses because of inability to afford healthcare, shelter and food.

After we gave the report, Nkechi and I wearily bade Obioma farewell and went to the dark outside restroom to freshen up. We removed the dirty aprons and fixed the caps. We washed our hands with some black soap and rain water from the night before. There were no plumbing or running tap water. I wanted to change into clean clothes, but Nkechi refused. She explained that by wearing our uniforms, the criminals would not bother us on our way home.

As we headed out to meet our motorcycle cabs, Nkechi warned me to stay on the unpaved path and to watch out for snakes and scorpions. I was horrified! I hate snakes and bugs. In fact, I hate anything that has the potential to bite! I started thinking of the pavements and the streetlights of New York!!! I started missing my car, the subways, and the Midtown sidewalks.

The ride home was an adventure. The motorcyclists charged more because it was dark. They kept swerving to avoid the potholes. Also, they rode without headlights. The moonlight lighted the way. Nkechi explained that this was to deter the armed burglars. At one point, we had to stop for almost thirty minutes because the driver thought that he saw armed robbers.

Nkechi cautioned me not to talk to anybody because they could detect that I came from overseas and kidnap me. I was so scared that I started shaking uncontrollably. Nkechi gave me one of her wonderful smiles and reassured me that our Nursing uniform would safeguard us from any crimes against us because most of the criminals would need medical care one day. I know she meant it as a joke, but I did not find it funny. I was not feeling safe at this point. I calmed down, but I made a mental note not to take the hospital security guards at my hospital for granted again!

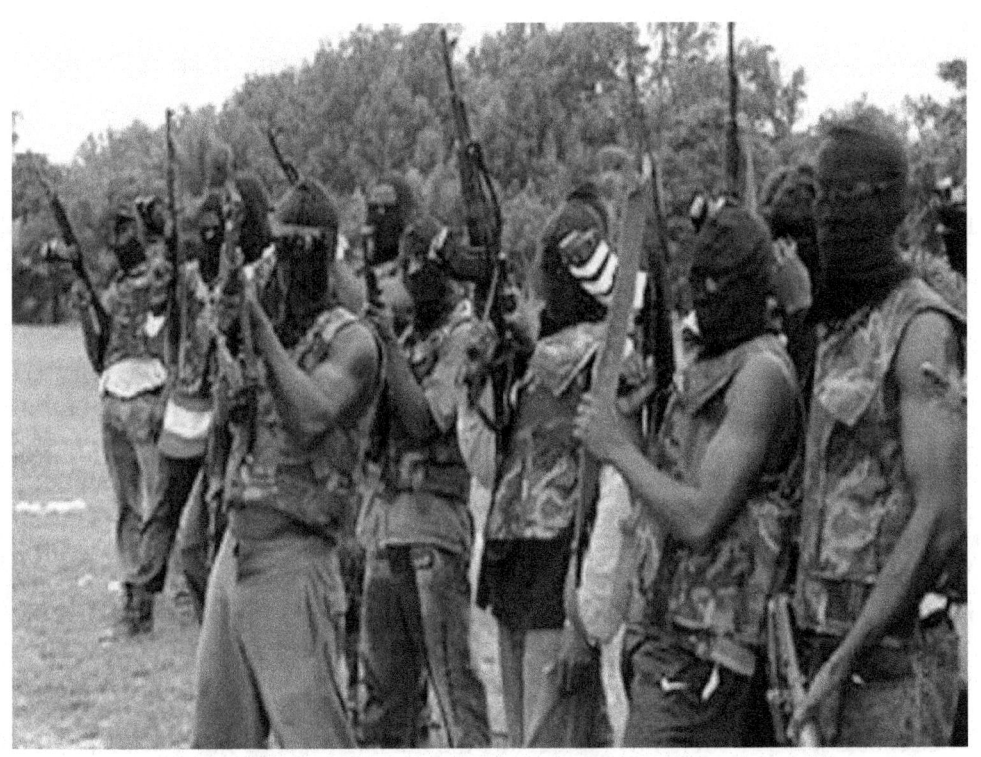

Courtesy of http://en.africatime.com - Notorious armed robbery gangs smashed

The crime rate in Nigeria could be attributed to the poverty in Nigeria. There is a high unemployment rate. Young Nigerian adults graduate from college without the prospect of getting any real jobs. Unlike the United States, there are no governmental social services to assist theses unemployed Nigerians. As mentioned above, the Nigerian government is corrupt and misappropriates the country's economy. Seeking ways to survive and to help their families, many young Nigerians will resort to criminal activities.

Reflection

By the time we got home, I was emotionally and physically fatigued! How could anybody live and work like this every day? I hugged Nkechi goodnight and thanked her for a memorable experience. I took a long hot shower and went into a dreamless sleep until 12 noon the next day. When I woke up, I realized that I had sores on the soles of my feet, a first-degree burn on the inside of my left leg, aching muscles and total exhaustion.

I went back to the bed waiting to fall back to sleep. I couldn't help thinking of my friend who had to do this every day to feed her family and to survive. There is no deliberate calling in sick, taking a mental health day or taking a vacation day to rest. If Nkechi, Chinyere or Obioma stayed away from work, they would not be paid. Nigerian Nurses' salaries are less than the minimum wage in the US.

Before I drifted off to sleep again, I thanked God that I was lucky to have that experience because I could now appreciate the nursing practice in the United States. Nurses trained in the United States need to be aware of the struggles of our counterparts practicing in other countries. United States nurses have to be thankful for some of the things we take for granted. We drive the latest or the newest cars. We work with up-to-date and sophisticated medical technology. We have endless days and nights of electricity. Our working environment is clean and safe. We have the ability to voice our opinions. The healthcare is regulated. Every time we need water, we could have clean running water and indoor plumbing. We could travel anywhere and anytime without fear of armed robbery. Our workplace and our patients are safe at all times.

Nowadays, when we are short of staff, or we have to go that extra mile to care for a patient, I no longer get angry because I think of Nkechi barely making ends meet to provide for her patients, for her family and herself. When I hear nurses complain about trivial issues such as having to go for continuing education classes or learning new skills, I wish that I could introduce them to Nkechi and to all other nurses struggling to keep their patients and their families alive.

Also, since nursing is mostly a female dominated profession, we have to be aware of issues that face women globally such as forced marriages, forced sex, female circumcision, inadequate birth control, unequal treatment and pay, inability to inherit from spouses, and treatment of women as second-class citizens.

Conclusion

As an immigrant to this country, I have always been fascinated with the culture of other people especially their approach to healthcare practices and decision making. I based my nursing practice on transcultural nursing.

According to the founder of this nursing theory, Madeleine Leininger, "To be culturally competent, the nurse needs to understand his/her own world views and those of the patient while avoiding stereotyping and misapplication of scientific knowledge. Cultural competence is obtaining cultural information and then applying that knowledge. This cultural awareness allows you to see the entire picture and improves the quality of care and health outcomes. Adapting to different cultural beliefs and practices requires flexibility and respect for others viewpoints. Cultural competence means actually to listen to the patient, to find out and learn about the patient's beliefs about health and illness. To provide the culturally appropriate care we need to know and to understand culturally influenced health behaviors (Leininger, 1991)".

To me, culture is not just about belief and habits of a particular race. Culture can also be about different religions, various units within a hospital and different way of life that is different from what is familiar. Using this theory, I have always learned to interact with other from different cultures by first doing self-examination about my personal prejudices and generalizations about the other person's culture. Then I will research the information about the culture especially their beliefs about life, health and decision making. After this, I will try to clarify any misconceptions that I have by asking the person or doing additional research about the culture. I empathize and actively listen to any intercultural communication.

Nurses need to be aware of these global issues that affect their counterparts all over the world.

Global nursing is not about transcultural nursing but about being cognizant of healthcare matters that affect people all over the world. With this knowledge, we will be able to provide sensitive, cultural care to our patients. Also, we will be able to empathize with our colleagues that are migrating to this country. This knowledge will be an immense assistance with the utilization of healthcare resources, practicing cost effective nursing, and appreciating the nursing practice in this country.

Bibliography

Echezona-Johnson, Chinazo. "Pregnancy in African cultures" https://www.
    academia.edu/10008232/Pregnancy_in_African_cultures

Echezona-Johnson, Chinazo. "SEXUAL TABOOS AND HIV/AIDS IN AFRICA"
    https://www.academia.edu/9986653/SEXUAL_TABOOS_AND_HIV_AID
    S_IN_AFRICA

Echezona-Johnson, Chinazo. "Maternal Pregnancy Risks in African Countries"
    https://www.academia.edu/22236542/Maternal_Pregnancy_Risks_in_Africa
    n_Countries

Echezona-Johnson, Chinazo. "Forms of Discrimination that Exist"https://
    www.academia.edu/13132078/Forms_of_Discrimination_that_Exist
    "Female genital mutilation", Geneva: World Health Organization, February
    2016.

"Female genital mutilation", Geneva: World Health Organization, February 2016.

Global future nurse. (n.d.). Retrieved from http://professional royalnurse.
    blogspot.com/

http://chukwudiiwuchukwu.blogspot.com/

Itoro E. Akpan-Iquot. "Traditional marriage in Nigeria: Polygamy". Migerian
    womenworld.com. Retrieved 21 November 2014

Leininger, M. (1991). Transcultural nursing: the study and practice field. . Imprint,
    38(2), 55-66.US, O. (2005, April 26 Tuesday). Common dreams. Retrieved
    July 11, 2009, from Common dreams.org:
    http://www.commondreams.org/headlines
    05/0426-10.htm

www.ingramcontent.com/pod-product-compliance
Lightning Source LLC
Chambersburg PA
CBHW070338190526
45169CB00005B/1952